Clinical Assessment

Survival Guide

Second Edition

Tracy Lapworth and
Deborah Cook

...eis Group

LONDON AND NEW YORK

Second edition published 2023

by Routledge
4 Park Square, Milton Park, Abingdon, Oxon OX14 4RN

and by Routledge
605 Third Avenue, New York, NY 10158

Routledge is an imprint of the Taylor & Francis Group, an informa business

First edition published by 2013

British Library Cataloguing-in-Publication Data
A catalogue record for this book is available from the British Library

Library of Congress Cataloging-in-Publication Data
Names: Lapworth, Tracy, 1964- author. I Cook, Deborah, 1964- author.
Title: Clinical assessment / Tracy Lapworth and Deborah Cook.
Description: Second edition. I Abingdon, Oxon ; New York, NY : Routledge, 2022. I Includes bibliographical references and index.
Identifiers: LCCN 2022021093 (print) I LCCN 2022021094 (ebook) I ISBN 9781032196855 (spiral bound) I ISBN 9781003260325 (ebook)
Subjects: LCSH: Nursing assessment.
Classification: LCC RT48 .L37 2022 (print) I LCC RT48 (ebook) I DDC 616.07/5--dc23/eng/20220816
LC record available at https://lccn.loc.gov/2022021093
LC ebook record available at https://lccn.loc.gov/2022021094

ISBN: 978-1-032-19685-5 (pbk)

ISBN: 978-1-003-26032-5 (ebk)

DOI: 10.4324/9781003260325

Typeset in Helvetica
by MPS Limited, Dehradun

contents

igures

Tables

introduction to the second edition

This book has been designed as a guide to assist you in the holistic health assessment of your patient. It will provide an overview of the principles of history taking and holistic health assessment. It has been updated to reflect the recent global challenges to health assessment because of the COVID-19 pandemic, including how we include BAME considerations and how we use our resources wisely to meet the growing demand on health services.

In addition to this book, you are strongly advised to read around the topics introduced; examples of useful resources are provided within each chapter.

Whether comprehensive or focused, assessment forms the basis of clinical decision making – every patient/client contact is an opportunity for assessment.

A health assessment comprises taking a health history and performing a physical examination, to collect both subjective and objective data. History taking collects subjective data, information that cannot be verified by anyone except the patient. The physical examination will collect objective data, e.g. listening to adventitious breath sounds.

This guide introduces the student to a structured format of history taking and to the factors involved in taking a comprehensive history. It introduces the four core physical

DOI: 10.4324/9781003260325-1

assessment skills: inspection, palpation, percussion and auscultation, and discusses how to document findings from history taking and physical examination in six of the major body systems.

The subject of mental health assessment is not covered within this book; however, this is an extremely important part of health assessment and therefore students are strongly advised to address this area as part of their continued development in holistic health assessment.

History taking

> In taking histories follow each line of thought, ask no leading questions. Never suggest. Give the patient's own words in the complaint.
> (from Osler, cited in Huth and Murray, 2000)

History taking is a vital part of the assessment process and helps to illustrate a truly holistic picture of the patient. A good health history can be said to provide 80% of the information needed for a diagnosis (Epstein et al., 2008).

SEQUENCE OF EVENTS IN HISTORY TAKING

1. Biographical data
2. Reason for seeking care (presenting complaint)
3. Present health/history of present illness
4. Past history
5. Family history
6. Personal and social history
7. Functional assessment or activities of daily living
8. Review of systems

TYPES OF HISTORY

- **Comprehensive** – includes all the areas discussed in this chapter and is therefore the more likely format used to give a complete picture of the patient
- **Focused** – the questions are driven by the presenting complaint, e.g. minor illness or injury. In this case,

DOI: 10.4324/9781003260325-2

information related to the presenting complaint and management may be all that is required

- **Emergency situations** – An ABCDE assessment (Resuscitation Council (UK), 2021) may be needed with a brief focused history where the patient is acutely unwell, e.g. sepsis
- **Preoperative assessment** – the focus is on past surgery and factors related to safe anaesthesia, e.g. respiratory and cardiac systems
- **Follow-up assessment** – the patient may be well known to the practitioner so history taking will be building on past information
- **Mental health assessment**
- **Nutritional assessment**

The last two forms of assessment are not addressed in this guide.

Note *It takes more skill to decide and have confidence not to ask questions. If in any doubt, ask rather than not!*

■ TIPS FOR OBTAINING A SUCCESSFUL HISTORY

- The information gained from history taking will depend greatly on your communication and questioning skills
- Introduce yourself and describe your role, explain the purpose of the interview and approximately how long it will take
- Gain consent from the patient to take the history. Please ensure they have mental capacity and cognitive ability
- Establish how the patient wishes to be addressed

Establish patient gender and how they identify themselves

- Discuss the presence of any other people present and if they are expected to participate
- Discuss confidentiality – the information you ascertain will be kept confidential within the healthcare team (unless the patient is a child or vulnerable adult and you suspect abuse; then you may need to share this information with other professionals)
- Remember the importance of non-verbal clues and body language
- Consider the use of touch – it may help to demonstrate understanding and can be therapeutic if culturally appropriate. You will need to assess whether there are any language or communication issues and whether assistance, e.g. an interpreter, is required

The mnemonic SOLER (Egan, 2001) can improve your listening skills:

S – Sit squarely facing the patient, although some prefer a slight angle

O – Open posture

L – Lean towards the patient

E – Eye contact

R – Relaxed approach

Note *Guidance from NHS England and the National Institute for Health and Care Excellence states clearly that face-to-face contact should be minimised in all settings during the recent COVID-19 pandemic. Remote video*

and telephone consultations between clinician and patient are increasingly introduced in some settings replacing face-to-face consultations. There are advantages to patients in relation ease of access and reduction of travel but may pose challenges in relation to communication and assessment.

As a consequence of COVID-19, healthcare workers undertaking assessments are often wearing PPE, which can also pose a significant challenge to building rapport due to the sense of disconnect and distraction created by the PPE, difficulty hearing what the patient or clinician is saying and loss of lip reading or visual cues.

■ TYPES OF QUESTION

Asking open-ended questions allows the patient to respond more freely and helps you to discover the real problem without leading or directing, e.g. 'What has brought you here to see me today?' Don't interrupt too soon, though – wait until the patient has finished answering this question!

Closed questions can be useful to establish specific facts but should be used carefully.

Table 1.1 Open-ended and closed questions

OPEN-ENDED	CLOSED
Used to open interview	Calls for specific information
Calls for long answers	Results in one- or two-word answers

able 1.1 (*Continued*)

OPEN-ENDED	CLOSED
Encourages feelings and ideas	Results in hard facts
Lets the patient express themselves	Limits rapport
Enhances rapport	Speeds up interview

Table 1.2 Aids to information gathering/ten traps of interviewing

AIDS TO INFORMATION GATHERING	TEN TRAPS OF INTERVIEWING
• **Facilitation** – use of expressions such as 'please go on' will demonstrate that you want the patient to continue • **Reflection** – use reflective comments to encourage the patient: 'yes I see that' • **Clarification** – useful when the information from the patient is vague, e.g. 'the pain is everywhere'; 'point	• **Providing false reassurance** – don't be tempted to reassure the patient that everything will be fine until you are sure of your facts • **Giving unwanted advice** – the patient may have lifestyle choices that may need addressing – choose the moment to discuss these carefully • **Using authority** • **Engaging in distancing** – be wary of barriers such as desks

(*Continued*)

Table 1.2 (Continued)

AIDS TO INFORMATION GATHERING	TEN TRAPS OF INTERVIEWING
to where the pain is on your body' • **Empathy** – listen to the total communication given by words, feelings and body language, and demonstrate that you are listening to the effect that the problem has on the patient's life • **Demonstrate interest** in the patient's feelings • **Interpretation** – restate the information the patient has given you to make sure that it is an accurate account	• **Using avoidance language** – death is a classic example: 'your father has moved on' • **Using jargon words** such as myocardial infarction and CVA • **Using leading questions** – 'you don't take drugs, do you?', 'the pain doesn't go down your arm, does it?' • **Talking too much** – don't underestimate the importance of silence • **Interrupting** – if you do this you may miss vital information • **Using why questions** – this can be quite accusatory

■ PRESENTING COMPLAINT

• Obtain a full description of the patient's main complaint
• Discover the sequence of symptom formation

Clarify and summarise symptoms and find out if there are any other major problems

- It is best to begin with a single sentence, e.g. *c/o abdominal pain for 3 days*
- Determine when the illness first began
- Describe symptoms in chronological order
- Obtain a detailed description of the symptoms: duration, onset, constant or sporadic, frequency, worsening or easing, any precipitating factors

Evaluating a symptom

Does the patient's condition indicate an emergency? An ABCDE assessment (Resuscitation Council (UK), 2021) will be needed.

Table 1.3 Does the patient's condition indicate an emergency?

NO	YES
Take a thorough history	Take a brief history
Thoroughly examine the patient	Perform a focused physical examination
Evaluate findings – are emergency signs present?	Evaluate findings – are emergency signs present?
Review your findings to consider possible causes	Intervene appropriately to stabilise the patient
Evaluate your findings and devise an appropriate plan of care	Review the patient's condition to consider possible causes (Morton, 1993)

Note When trying to establish and explore the presenting complaint, it is best to start with an open-ended question and use the patient's own words where possible. Most patients will tell you the problem within 1–2 minutes if uninterrupted (Snadden et al., 2005).

Exploring the presenting complaint

There are various mnemonics to help explore the presenting complaint to help ensure that pertinent data is not missed.

PQRSTU (Morton, 1993)

P Provocative or palliative – does anything make the problem worse or better? Has treatment helped? Make sure you ask the questions separately

Q Quantity or quality – what does the symptom feel like? How does it affect normal life? If there are secretions involved, e.g. sputum, how much is the patient expectorating?

R Region or radiation – where in the body does the symptom occur? Does it spread anywhere else? Does anything else happen with it?

S Severity/symptoms – how severe is the problem? Are there any other associated symptoms? Use a scale, e.g. 1–10. Is it getting worse or better?

T Timing – when did the symptom start? Was it a sudden or gradual onset? How often does it occur? How long does it last? Is it getting worse?

U Understanding – does the patient have any thoughts on what may be causing the symptom?

OLD CARTS (Seidel et al., 2003)

Onset – when did the symptom start? Was it a sudden or gradual onset? How often does it occur?

Location – where in the body does the symptom occur? Does it spread anywhere else?

Duration – how often does the symptom occur? How long does it last? Is it getting worse?

Characteristics – what does the symptom feel like, look like or sound like?

Associated and aggravating factors – do you have any other symptoms at the moment that seem to be linked to this one? Is there anything that makes it worse?

Relieving factors/radiation – does anything make it better? Does it radiate anywhere else?

Treatment – what treatments have you tried? Have they helped?

Severity – how severe is the symptom? Use a scale, e.g. 1–10. Is it getting worse or better?

CLIENT OUTCOMES (Rhoads, 2006)

Character – what does the symptom feel like, look like or sound like? How severe is the symptom? Use a scale, e.g. 1–10. Is it getting worse or better?

Location – where in the body does the symptom occur? Does it spread anywhere else?

Impact – what effect does the symptom have on the patient's daily life?

Expectation – what does the patient expect from the consultation?

Neglect/abuse – are there any signs of physical and emotional neglect or abuse?

Timing – when did the symptom start? Was it a sudden or gradual onset? How often does it occur? How long does it last? Is it getting worse?

Other – does the patient have any other symptoms at the moment that seem to be linked to this one?

Understanding – does the patient have any thoughts on what may be causing the symptom?

Treatment – what treatments have the patient tried? Have they helped?

Complementary – any use of complementary therapies?

Options – are there options for care for the patient, e.g. advance directives?

Modulating factors – e.g. aggravate/alleviate – does anything make the problem worse or better? Make sure you ask the questions separately

Exposure – infection/toxic – has there been any exposure to infectious agents?

Spirituality – what are the patient's spiritual needs or beliefs?

Note Include:
* pertinent positives and negatives
* the patient's response to the symptoms
* the effect the problem has on the patient's life

The data flows spontaneously from the patient, but the task of organising it is yours!

■ PAST MEDICAL HISTORY

It may be useful to start with an open question, such as: 'Tell me about any problems you have had in the past with our health.' You may then need to use the following prompts.

Childhood illnesses

- Measles, mumps, chicken pox, etc.
- Any chronic childhood illness

Enquire about adult illness in four areas.

Table 1.4 Four areas of illness

MEDICAL	PSYCHIATRIC
Exclude illness such as diabetes, stroke, hypertension, asthma, epilepsy, heart disease and cancer. Any hospitalisations	Illness, hospitalisation, treatments
SURGICAL	**OBSTETRIC/GYNAECOLOGICAL**
Dates and types of operation	Obstetric history, menstrual history, contraception, sexual function

Drug history

A full medication history must be taken. A complete list of current medication should be made:

- Prescribed
- Homeopathic
- Over the counter

- Recreational
- From any other sources, e.g. Internet, family

Note *The patient's GP practice may need to be contacted.*
Concordance with medication should be checked; if
non-concordance is present, explore the reasons.

Allergies

Drugs

- Are there any allergies to drugs? Record the severity and nature of the reaction
- What happened?
- What were the symptoms?
- Was hospital treatment required?

Environment and foodstuffs

- Any allergies to pollen, foodstuffs, pets, bee stings, etc.? Record the severity and nature of the reaction
- What happened?
- What were the symptoms?
- Was hospital treatment required?

Family history

Asking the patient about the health of their family could provide important information relating to risk factors for disease.

- Parents: are they alive or deceased? If dead, from what cause? At what age?

Siblings: are they fit and well?

Close family members, i.e. spouse or children

Is there any history of:

- diabetes
- epilepsy
- mental disorders
- heart problems
- high blood pressure
- stroke
- cancer
- asthma
- thyroid problems

Common disorders expressed in families

- Ischaemic heart disease
- Diabetes mellitus
- Hypertension
- Myopia
- Alcoholism
- Depression
- Osteoporosis
- Cancer: bowel, ovarian, breast

Personal history

The aim is to understand how the patient's illness relates to his or her personal circumstances and personality.

Ask general questions to include: family, work, hobbies, eating out, exposure to infection, housing, smoking, alcohol, drugs, travel abroad, workplace hazards, carers, home help, social prescribing, belief system, financial issues.

Travel-related risks (Epstein et al., 2008)

- Viral diseases: e.g. COVID-19, hepatitis A, B, C, yellow fever, rabies, polio
- Bacterial diseases: e.g. salmonella, shigella, E. coli, cholera, meningitis, tetanus, Lyme's disease
- Parasites: e.g. malaria, schistosomiasis

Smoking history

- Ascertain whether the patient, or anyone in the household, smokes
- If the person is an ex-smoker, find out when he or she stopped
- If a smoker, has the patient ever tried to stop? Would he or she like to?
- The more the patient smokes or has smoked, the greater the risk and therefore a useful classification is pack years:

Pack years : 1 pack = 20 cigarettes

$$\frac{\text{Number of packs of cigarettes smoked daily} \times \text{number of years of smoking}}{20}$$

If the person smokes 20 a day, the pack years will always be the same as the number of years for which they have smoked.

Ascertain whether the patient, or anyone in the household uses vapes, explore the frequency, nature and type of vape solution.

Alcohol

- Start questioning with an open question: 'Do you drink any alcohol? What do you like drinking?'
- Ascertain glass size, amount and habit – if the patient drinks every night, do they drink more at the weekend?
- Patients may feel uncomfortable about disclosing the true amount of alcohol and therefore it may be useful to overestimate, e.g. 'so do you drink six gin and tonics a night?' The patient may then admit that it is four
- If you suspect the patient's alcohol consumption is hazardous, then there are various screening systems that can be applied

CAGE screening system (Bickley, 2020)

- Have you ever thought that you need to **cut down**?
- Have you ever felt **annoyed** by criticism about your drinking?
- Have you ever felt **guilty** about drinking?
- Have you ever taken a drink first thing in the morning **(eye-opener)** to steady your nerves or for a hangover?

If the patient says yes to two or more of these questions, there may be a problem.

Audit PC screening tool

Table 1.5 Audit PC screening tool

QUESTIONS	SCORING SYSTEM					YOUR SCORE
	0	1	2	3	4	
How often do you have a drink containing alcohol?	Never	Monthly or less	2–4 times per month	2–3 times per week	4+ times per week	
How many units of alcohol do you drink on a typical day when you are drinking?	1–2	3–4	5–6	7–8	10+	
How often during the last year have you found that you were not able to stop drinking once you had started?	Never	Less than monthly	Monthly	Weekly	Daily or almost daily	
How often during the last year have you failed to do what was normally expected from you because of your drinking?	Never	Less than monthly	Monthly	Weekly	Daily or almost daily	

ble 1.5 (Continued)

UESTIONS	SCORING SYSTEM					YOUR SCORE
	0	1	2	3	4	
as a relative r friend, octor or other ealth worker een concerned bout your rinking or uggested that ou cut down?	No		Yes, but not in the last year		Yes, during the last year	

oring: A total of 5+ indicates increasing or higher risk drinking; an overall total re of 5 or above is AUDIT-PC-positive.

Drugs

- Ask about recreational drugs
- This may be a sensitive area for questions, but the effects on physical and mental health and drug interaction makes this information very important
- If the patient admits to drug use, ascertain which drugs they actually take by name: cocaine, heroin, marijuana – there may be other street names with which you are not familiar, so try to acquire these names, too
- Ascertain quantity – you can apply the CAGE questionnaire to drugs as well as to alcohol

Sexual history

This may be a sensitive area for questions. Start with an open question:

- Have you any sexual concerns?
- Explore areas such as possible pregnancy
- Current sexual partner – male or female?
- Methods of contraception
- Previous history of sexually transmitted infections (STIs)

Functional assessment

Asking these questions will provide you with important information about the effect of the symptom on activities of daily living of the patient and potential problems with general health. Begin with general enquiries:

- Appetite and diet – any change?
- Weight – any unexpected weight loss or gain?
- Fatigue
- Fever or chills
- Night sweats
- Aches or pains
- Rashes
- Lumps or bumps

Review of systems

The review of systems will help to provide a complete overview of the patient's health. It can also act as a safety net to ensure that any important issues are not overlooked. You may warn the patient that you will be asking questions that seem unrelated to their symptoms but that these are important to gain a true picture of their health.

Start from head and work to toe (Bickley, 2020):

- General
- Skin
- Head, eyes, ears, nose, throat (HEENT)

- Neck
- Breasts
- Respiratory
- Cardiovascular
- Gastrointestinal
- Genitourinary
- Peripheral vascular
- Musculoskeletal
- Neurological
- Endocrine
- Psychiatric

Note *If a system has already been explored as the presenting complaint, it does not have to be addressed again.*

Patient perspective

- What do you think the problem is caused by?
- What are your main worries?
- What are you expecting to happen following the consultation?
- Any questions?

Table 1.6 History-taking summary

	AREAS TO EXPLORE
Demographics	Age, gender and type of employment
Onset	Gradual onset will offer different differential diagnoses compared

(Continued)

Table 1.6 (*Continued*)

	AREAS TO EXPLORE
	to sudden-onset conditions. Has the patient been affected by this problem at other times?
Location	Location of problem, describe anatomically
Duration	How often is the problem occurring? Has this changed? How long do the episodes last and has this changed?
Characteristics	How does the patient describe the problem?
Associated symptoms	For example: nausea, vomiting, weight loss, itching, swelling, redness, systemic illness For each presenting complaint there will be specific associated symptoms that need to be explored
Aggravating factors	Is there anything that makes the problem worse?
Relieving factors	Is there anything that makes the problem better?
Temporal factors	What does the patient think is the problem? What concerns them the most?

able 1.6 (*Continued*)

	AREAS TO EXPLORE
Severity	How does the problem affect the patient's activities of daily living?
Medications	Prescription-only medicine, over the counter, homeopathic, recreational; any others?
Allergies	To medications, foods or environmental factors. How severe is the reaction?
Past medical history	Any major diseases, e.g. diabetes, epilepsy, thromboembolic disease, cardiovascular disease, malignancy, etc.
Family history	Any familial major diseases: parents, siblings, children
Social history	Living arrangements, occupation, exposure to toxins, recent travel abroad, smoking history, use of alcohol, sexual history, hobbies
Review of systems	HEENT: hearing, sight, swallowing, speech Neurological: fits, faints or 'funny turns' Cardiac: chest pain, palpitations Respiratory: breathing problems, wheeze, cough

(*Continued*)

Table 1.6 (*Continued*)

	AREAS TO EXPLORE
	Gastrointestinal: bowel habit, weight, appetite Genitourinary: sexual health, urinary symptoms Musculoskeletal: gait, weight-bearing, muscle tone Endocrine: normal skin condition, mood changes, sensation to heat Psychological: any existing mental health issues, anxiety, mood

The history taking should lead to the following:
- An approximate diagnosis
- A rapport between patient and practitioner
- A picture of the patient as a whole
- A guide to which areas to examine in the physical assessment
- After conclusion of the consultation, formulation of a plan of care for the patient

The following mnemonic can help to identify potential causes of the patient's problem.

VITAMINS C DEF: cause of the symptom(s)

- **V**ascular, e.g. myocardial infarct
- **I**nfectious
- **T**raumatic

Autoimmune/allergic
Metabolic, e.g. diabetes
Idiopathic/iatrogenic, e.g. drug interaction
Neoplastic
Substance abuse and psychiatric
Congenital
Degenerative
Endocrine
Functional

SUMMARY

The success and quality of the history depends on the communication skills of the health care professional, which may be more challenging in areas highlighted such as telephone and video consultations and wearing of PPE.

A comprehensive health history should reflect awareness of the need for cultural and spiritual assessment and appreciation of the diversity of patients to include gender, ethnicity, cognitive ability, mental health and social needs (social prescribing) in line with The NHS Long Term Plan goals (NHS, 2019).

■ USEFUL RESOURCES

Bickley, L.S. (2020) *Bates' Guide to Physical Examination and History Taking*, Wolters Kluwer Health, Amsterdam.

Buck, D., Ewbank, L. (2020) What is social prescribing? Available at https://www.kingsfund.org.uk/publications/social-prescribing

Centres for Disease Control and Prevention. Available at https://www.cdc.gov/std/treatment/ SexualHistory.htm

Dean, E. (2020) Remote nursing consultations: How to get them right. *Nursing Standard*. Available at https://rcni.com/nursing-standard/newsroom/analysis/remote-nursing-consultations-how-to-get-them-right-16136

Egan, G. (2001) *The Skilled Helper: A problem management and opportunity development approach to helping*, 7th edn., Wadsworth Publishing Company, Kentucky.

Epstein, O., Perkin, G.D., Cookson, J., Watt, I.S., Rakhit, R., Robins, A., Hornett, G.A.W. (2008) *Clinical Examination*, 4th edn., Mosby, Edinburgh.

Huth, E.J., Murray, T.J. (eds.) (2000) *Medicine in Quotations: Views of health and disease through the ages*, American College of Physicians, Philadelphia.

Interviewing and the Health History. Available at https://usermanual.wiki/Document/BatesChapter2.1293603966.pdf

McNeill, A., Brose, L.S., Calder, R., Simonavicius, E., Robson, D. (2021) *Vaping in England: An evidence update including vaping for smoking cessation, February 2021: a report commissioned by PHE*. London: PHE. Available at https://www.gov.uk/government/publications/vaping-in-england-evidence-update-february-2021/vaping-in-england-2021-evidence-update-summary

Morton, P. (1993) *Health Assessment in Nursing*, 2nd edn., Springhouse, Pennsylvania.

NHS England (2019) *The NHS Long Term Plan*. Available at https://www.longtermplan.nhs.uk/wp-content/uploads/2019/08/nhs-long-term-plan-version-1.2.pdf

National Healthcare National HR Directorate (2020) Communication skills for staff wearing personal protective equipment (PPE). Available at https://www.hse.ie/eng/about/our-health-service/healthcare-communication/nhcp-communication-skills-for-staff-wearing-personal-protective-equipment-ppe.pdf

Resuscitation Council (UK) (2021). Available at https://www.resus.org.uk/library/2021-resuscitation-guidelines/adult-basic-life-support-guidelines

Rhoads, J. (2006) *Advanced Health Assessment and Diagnostic Reasoning*, Lippincott, Wilkins, & Williams, Philadelphia.

Royal College of Nursing (2020) Having courageous conversations by telephone or video during the COVID-19 pandemic. Available at https://www.rcn.org.uk/Professional-Development/publications/rcn-courageousconversations-covid-19-uk-pub-009-236

Seidel, H., Ball, J., Dains, J., Benedict, G.W. (2003) *Mosby's Guide to Physical Examination*, 5th edn., Mosby, St Louis.

Snadden, D., Lang, R., Masterson, G., Colledge, N. (2005) History taking. In: Douglas, G., Nicol, F., Robertson, C. (eds.) *Macleod's Clinical Examination*, 11th edn, Churchill Livingstone, Edinburgh.

2 General assessment

- The physical examination of the patient will generally follow the history taking as this will direct which system to examine to prove or disprove a potential diagnosis
- Use a systematic approach
- The results from the examination, together with the history, will contribute to the bigger picture of the patient's health as a whole
- The physical examination starts by observation of the patient and forming a general impression of the state of their health

■ OBSERVING THE PATIENT

Initial assessment

In an emergency with an acutely ill patient, the ABCDE assessment structure should be followed (Resuscitation Council (UK), 2021).

Airway
Breathing
Circulation
Disability – assessing conscious level using the AVPU tool: **A**lert, responds to **V**oice, responds to **P**ain, **U**nconscious. Pupil reactions and blood glucose monitoring is also recommended
Exposure – look at the whole body, including the skin, any wounds or temperature abnormalities

DOI: 10.4324/9781003260325-3

he patient should also be assessed for the risk of sepsis
ising the NEWS2 scoring system on page 30 (https://www.
cplondon.ac.uk/projects/outputs/national-early-warning-
score-news-2) (https://www.nice.org.uk/guidance/NG51).

Emergency treatment plans should be administered and
a more in-depth assessment can be undertaken once the
patient has been stabilised.

SOME TEAMS (Rushforth, 2009)

- **S**ymmetry – are his face and body symmetrical?
- **O**ld – does he look his age?
- **M**entation – is he alert or confused?
- **E**xpression – does he look ill or in pain or anxious?
- **T**runk – what is his body type: lean or obese?
- **E**xtremities – are his fingers clubbed? Does he have any oedema or joint swelling?
- **A**ppearance – is he clean and appropriately dressed?
- **M**ovement – are his posture, gait and coordination normal?
- **S**peech – is his speech relaxed, strong, appropriate?

Note *There may be clues around the patient that contribute to the picture, e.g. inhalers, glyceryl trinitrate spray and sputum pot.*

■ VITAL SIGNS

The recording of a full and accurate set of vital signs is extremely important.

- Temperature, pulse, respirations, blood pressure (TPRBP), oxygen saturation and capillary refill
- Height and weight

Figure 2.1 The NEWS scoring system

Physiological parameter	Score						
	3	2	1	0	1	2	3
Respiration rate (per minute)	≤8		9–11	12–20		21–24	≥25
SpO₂ Scale 1 (%)	≤91	92–93	94–95	≥96			
SpO₂ Scale 2 (%)	≤83	84–85	86–87	88–92 / ≥93 on air	93–94 on oxygen	95–96 on oxygen	≥97 on oxygen
Air or oxygen?		Oxygen		Air			
Systolic blood pressure (mmHg)	≤90	91–100	101–110	111–219			≥220
Pulse (per minute)	≤40		41–50	51–90	91–110	111–130	≥131
Consciousness				Alert			CVPU
Temperature (°C)	≤35.0		35.1–36.0	36.1–38.0	38.1–39.0	≥39.1	

◀ EXAMINATION CHECKLIST

Introduce yourself, explain what the examination entails and gain verbal consent

Ensure that you have the necessary equipment, e.g. stethoscope, tendon hammer

▶ Ensure that you have privacy for the patient to undress and you maintain patient dignity

▶ If the patient is accompanied, ensure that you have ascertained whether the patient would wish the other person to stay or leave the room

● Be sensitive to cultural needs

Note   *The patient is historically examined from the right side. All examination techniques are designed using this approach.*

◀ THE EXAMINATION

The examination framework is based around the following techniques:

• **Inspection** – looking – observing for colour, symmetry, size, movement
• **Palpation** – this requires touching the patient, applying varying degrees of pressure to provide information. Tender areas are always palpated last. Gloves must be worn if there is the potential to encounter body fluids
• **Percussion** – this involves tapping the patient's body quickly with your fingers to elicit sounds. It may identify organs and whether they contain fluid or air. It requires a skilful ear and takes practice

Percussion sounds

Table 2.1 Percussion sounds

SOUND	QUALITY	LOCATION	SOURCE
Tympany	Drum-like, musical	Over enclosed air	Air in bowel
Resonance	Hollow, clear	Over air-filled areas that are partially solid	Normal lung
Hyper-resonance	Booming and hollow	Over large quantities of air	Lung with emphysema
Dullness	Thud-like and muffled	Over solid tissue	Liver, heart, spleen
Flatness	Flat and stony dull	Over dense tissue	Muscle, bone

- **Auscultation** – this involves listening for sounds with a stethoscope to determine presence or absence of sound and quality and nature of sound. It is generally performed at the end except in the examination of the abdomen. The head of the stethoscope has two surfaces: the bell and the diaphragm. The bell detects low sounds, the diaphragm high: bell-low, di-high! When using the stethoscope, the diaphragm needs to be pressed firmly on the skin; when using the bell, it needs to be placed lightly on the skin to form a seal. The tubing of the stethoscope should be 38 cm at its maximum length and have snug ear plugs that need to point towards the nose when in place. It will also have both a diaphragm and bell or the two will be integrated

Note Tips for successful auscultation
  - *Peace and quiet*
  - *Listen under clothes not over them – skin contact*
  - *Wet the chest hairs to restrict crackles*
  - *Warm the stethoscope head in your clean hand*
  - *Do not forget infection control – clean the ear plugs, bell and diaphragm with alcohol or chlorhexidine before and after each use*

For most of the main body systems, start by examining the hands, eyes and mouth. It is useful to develop a systematic approach and starting by examining the hands begins to introduce touch in a non-threatening way.

Skin

This is the first part of the patient you can see, so can give you some vital clues as to the wellness of the patient. Note the:
- Colour
- Temperature
- Turgidity
- Any rashes – see Chapter 3

Hands

Observe the hands and feel their warmth, observe for:
- Cold – low cardiac output, hypothyroidism

- Warmth – high cardiac output, CO_2 retention
- Cold and sweaty – sympathetic drive

Nails

Note presence of nails on all digits, observe for:
- Bitten – stress/anxiety related
- Blue tinges – may be difficult to detect in dark skin – peripheral cyanosis
- Leukonychia – white nails: albumin deficiency
- Koilonychia – spoon-shaped: iron deficiency
- Splinter haemorrhages can be a result of trauma, arteritis or subacute bacterial endocarditis (SBE)
- Osler's nodes – SBE
- Clubbing – loss of nail bed angle – see below

Figure 2.2 Nails

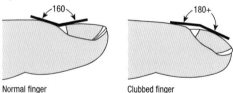

Normal finger   Clubbed finger

Causes of clubbing

- Lung disease: pyogenic (abscess), bronchial carcinoma, fibrosing alveolitis
- Heart disease: congenital heart disease, SBE
- Gastrointestinal: cirrhosis, ulcerative colitis, Crohn's disease

Palms

Erythema – can be normal, or CO_2 retention, chronic liver disease and pregnancy

Dupuytren's contractures – thickening of palmar fascia in little and ring fingers. Can indicate heavy alcohol and smoking habits

- Joint swelling – symmetrical in rheumatoid arthritis, asymmetrical in osteoarthritis and gout

Eyes

Look at both eyes – note any issues with the following.

Sclera

- Yellowness – liver disease, jaundice
- Blueness – in brittle bone disease
- Pale lower lid (regardless of skin colour) – anaemia, haemoglobin (Hb) < 9 g/dl

Cornea

- White bands – hypercholesterolaemia
- Xanthelasma – raised yellow lesions caused by the build-up of cholesterol
- Corneal arcus – a thin grey ring of lipids around the cornea

Mouth

Look at the tongue, teeth and mucous membranes, note any:

- Blue tongue – central cyanosis, severe COPD or cardiac shunt
- Dry tongue – dehydration or mouth breathing
- Bleeding or swollen gums – poor nutrition, poor dental care
- Red tonsils – see Chapter 4
- Breath odour – ketones in diabetic ketoacidosis, alcohol, hepatic fetor in liver failure

Lymph nodes

Examining the lymph nodes is part of most systems examinations and involves inspecting and palpating.

Figure 2.3 Lymph nodes

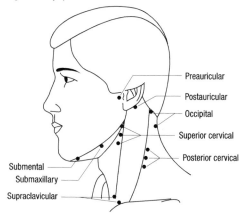

Preauricular

Postauricular

Occipital

Superior cervical

Posterior cervical

Submental

Submaxillary

Supraclavicular

he groups of lymph nodes accessible for examination are
the head and neck.

Enlarged nodes are usually visible, particularly if there is
asymmetrical enlargement

Infection may produce redness and inflammation

On palpation, normal nodes should not be felt

Malignancy may produce hard and irregular nodes

Raised nodes due to infection may be painful to palpate
and feel rubbery

◼ SUMMARY

A general assessment is the start point for a physical
examination; be logical, ensure your patient's safety,
comfort and dignity. Be sensitive to cultural issues and
aware that in the BAME population, anomalies may not be
as easily visible. This part of the examination develops
your rapport with the patient and introduces the element
of touch, so it is important to make a good first
impression.

◼ USEFUL RESOURCES

Bates Visual Guide to Physical Examination. Available at
https://batesvisualguide.com/
British Medical Journal Learning. Available at https://new-
learning.bmj.com/
Geeky Medics. Available at. https://geekymedics.com/
GP Notebook. Available at https://gpnotebook.com/en-gb/
Mind the Gap. Available at https://www.blackandbrownskin.
co.uk/mindthegap

National Institute of Health and Care Excellence (2021) COVID-19 Rapid Guideline: Managing COVID-19. Available at https://www.nice.org.uk/guidance/ng191/chapter/Recommendations

Resuscitation Council (UK) (2021). Available at https://www.resus.org.uk/library/2021-resuscitation-guidelines/adult-basic-life-support-guidelines

Rushforth, H. (2009) *Assessment Made Incredibly Easy!* Lippincott, Williams, & Wilkins, London.

Examination of the skin

Figure 3.1 Cross-section of the skin

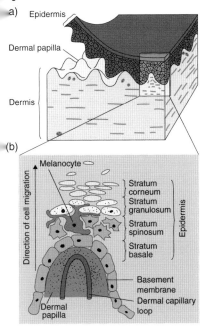

(a)

Epidermis

Dermal papilla

Dermis

(b)

Melanocyte

Direction of cell migration

Stratum corneum
Stratum granulosum
Stratum spinosum
Stratum basale

Epidermis

Basement membrane
Dermal capillary loop

Dermal papilla

DOI: 10.4324/9781003260325-4

The skin is the largest organ in the body and has a host of functions to maintain homeostasis. It is the part of the body that is exposed to the traumas of everyday life and is often the first area to give an indication of underlying disease. Examination of the skin includes both the hair and the nails.

Note Be sensitive in your approach; patients may be very aware of how their skin appears to others and an indication of the patient's psychological wellbeing may be given by their level of self-care and presentation.

- An ABCDE assessment (Resuscitation Council (UK), 2021) may be needed before examination continues – an urticarial rash may be the first sign of anaphylaxis
- Not all sick children/adolescents have a rash
- Skin colour and texture has many variations that are normal
- Skin and nail problems may be an indicator of underlying systemic disease
- Be aware of verbal and non-verbal cues
- Investigate the problem with a holistic health history: refer to Table 1.6
- Associated symptoms to explore are exposure to chemicals, nausea, vomiting, itching, swelling, redness and systemic illness
- Be aware of red flag markers – changes to moles, hair loss, new rashes, changes from normal
- Be safe – use gloves and aprons, and be aware of infection control

EXAMINATION

at all possible, examine the patient in natural light after aining a comprehensive history.

nspection

Compare the patient's normal areas to the affected areas and note the following:

- Colour of skin – pallor, cyanosis, jaundice and erythema may indicate systemic illness
- Uniformity of skin colour
- Rashes – noting the type and distribution of lesions
- Presence of wounds – old or new, scars, evidence of previous surgery
- Presence of petechiae – these may indicate systemic disease
- Any nail abnormalities – clubbing, splinter haemorrhages, fungal infection, colour of nails, nicotine staining
- Shape of nails – presence on all digits
- Thickness of nails
- Hair – hirsutism or alopecia may indicate hormonal imbalances; note the pattern of distribution

Palpate

Be aware that infection control measures may be necessary and note the following:

- Skin turgidity – this gives an indication of the patient's level of hydration
- Skin texture – rough dry skin may indicate hypothyroidism or psoriasis
- Any presence of oedema – may indicate underlying disease
- Level of moisture – skin is usually relatively dry

- Skin temperature – use the back of your hands and check bilaterally
- Location of any raised lesions

■ LESION CLASSIFICATION

Figure 3.2 Classification of lesions

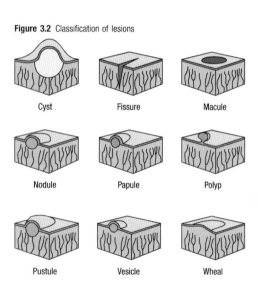

Cyst

Fissure

Macule

Nodule

Papule

Polyp

Pustule

Vesicle

Wheal

Table 3.1 Classification of lesions

LESION	DESCRIPTION	EXAMPLE
Cyst	Closed sac, with distinct membrane. May contain air, fluid or semi-solid material, but not pus, as this would be described as an abscess	Baker's cyst Chalazion
Fissure	Crack-like lesion that extends at least to the dermis	Athlete's foot
Macule	A circumscribed change in colour or consistency without elevation above surrounding skin, less than 1 cm in size. Larger than 1 cm is known as a patch	Freckles
Nodule	As for a papule but greater than 1 cm	Fibroma
Polyp	A small benign tumour that usually develops where the skin forms creases	Skin tag
Pustule	A papule filled with pus	Acne
Vesicle	A circumscribed, raised lesion, of less than 1cm in diameter containing clear serous fluid	Early chicken pox
Wheal	Raised circumscribed oedematous plaques, usually	Allergic reaction

(Continued)

Table 3.1 (*Continued*)

LESION	DESCRIPTION	EXAMPLE
	pink or pale, can be itchy and transient. Wheals that merge together to form a larger rash are known as urticaria	

■ PATTERNS OF LESION DISTRIBUTION

Table 3.2 Patterns of lesion distribution

NAME	DESCRIPTION
Discrete	Individual separate distinct lesions
Scattered	Lesions spread across the body
Localised	Lesions involved in only a selected part of the body
Annular	Lesions arranged in a single circle
Reticular	Net-like clusters of lesions
Grouped	Lesions that are clustered together in one or more groups; also called clusters
Polycyclic	A number of annular lesions arranged in multiple circles; also called gyrated
Linear	Lesions arranged in a line
Arciform	Lesions form arcs, curves or twists

Table 3.2 (*Continued*)

NAME	DESCRIPTION
Confluent	Multiple lesions that blend together so that individual lesions cannot be seen or palpated
Dermatomal	Lesions distributed along neurocutaneous dermatomes

ABCDE ASSESSMENT OF MALIGNANT MELANOMA

Malignant melanoma is the least common, but most serious, skin cancer, with 16,744 new cases in the UK in 2016–2018 (Cancer Research UK, 2022). Early recognition and diagnosis allows prompt treatment to commence. An ABCDE approach has been developed that aids diagnosis of this condition:

Asymmetry of the lesion border
Border irregularity
Colour of lesion varies with shades of tan, brown or black, and, possibly, red, blue or white
Diameter is typically greater than 6 mm or ¼ inch
Evolution, elevated or enlarging lesion

If any of these indicators are noted, the patient should be referred as soon as possible to a specialist.

■ SUMMARY

Despite being the largest organ in the body, the skin is sometimes overlooked. It can be the first area to indicate underlying disease. Gaining a holistic history will aid diagnosis. It may be difficult to diagnose the condition, but attempt to describe it and indicate the distribution on a diagram, which will allow concise referrals. Consider different presentations with BAME patients and the range of 'normal' findings.

■ USEFUL RESOURCES

Cancer Research UK (2022). Available at https://www.cancerresearchuk.org/health-professional/cancer-statistics/statistics-by-cancer-type/melanoma-skin-cancer

Mind the Gap. Available at https://www.blackandbrownskin.co.uk/mindthegap

Resuscitation Council (UK) (2021). Available at https://www.resus.org.uk/library/2021-resuscitation-guidelines/adult-basic-life-support-guidelines

Examination of the head, eyes, ears, nose and throat (HEENT) system

An examination of the HEENT system includes the head, eyes, ears, nose and throat.

Note *Be sensitive in your approach; the face gives away many facets of a person's physical and psychological health.*

- You may need an ABCDE assessment (Resuscitation Council (UK), 2021) and give analgesia before you can proceed with your examination
- HEENT presentations may be indicators of systemic disease; refer to Table 1.6 to gain a holistic history
- The age, gender and occupation of the patient may influence both probability of a diagnosis and compliance with treatment plans
- Associated symptoms for exploration: nausea, vomiting, change in vision, hearing, voice changes, headache, epistaxis, tinnitus, vertigo, temperature, changes to the sense of taste or smell and exposure to chemicals
- Be aware of red flag markers such as headache, vision changes, diplopia, changes in hearing, tinnitus, vertigo, epistaxis, hoarseness, swollen glands or goitre

■ EXAMINATION

Head and face

Observe the quantity, distribution and texture of the hair, palpate the scalp for lumps and lesions, note the skull

DOI: 10.4324/9781003260325-5

shape, size and contour, facial symmetry, skin colour and condition, and note any rashes or red areas. Tap the sinuses to elicit any tenderness.

Eyes

Compare eyes, check and record visual acuity. Where possible, use a slit lamp to examine the eyes. Observe all the eye structures: orbit, eyebrows, lids, lashes, conjunctiva, sclera, cornea, pupil, iris, lens, anterior chamber and retina. Note the symmetry, shape, size and presence of foreign bodies. Note pupil reaction to light, check visual fields and range and equality of ocular movements: 1. right, 2. up/right, 3. down/right, 4. left, 5. up/left, 6. down/left, and, finally, convergence.

Ears

Use an auroscope with a bright light to conduct this examination. Visualise the unaffected side first and compare with the affected side. Observe the auricle, note shape and

Figure 4.1 Right eardrum

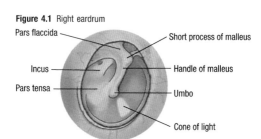

Pars flaccida

Short process of malleus

Incus

Handle of malleus

Pars tensa

Umbo

Cone of light

ize and palpate for swellings and any tenderness in the mastoid area. Straighten the external auditory meatus by firmly pulling the auricle up and slightly out. Look at the canal and tympanic membrane.

Nose

Use a bright light and speculum to conduct this part of the examination. Inspect the external and internal structures: look for symmetry, redness, polyps, swellings and bleeding. Look at the septum. Palpate the nares for nodules and firmness and check the patency of each.

Mouth, pharynx and neck

Inspect the lips, oral mucosa, gums, teeth, roof of the mouth, tongue, tonsils and neck, looking for symmetry, colour, swellings and deformities. Also note oral odour. Palpate the lymph nodes, trachea position and thyroid gland noting any abnormalities.

■ SUMMARY

A holistic history will guide the clinical examination and suggest a probable clinical diagnosis. As the face is a key element in how we communicate with the world, it is vital that the health professional deals with these patients with sensitivity and empathy.

■ USEFUL RESOURCES

ENT examination:
https://www.nei.nih.gov/learn-about-eye-health/eye-conditions-and-diseases

https://www.ole.bris.ac.uk/bbcswebdav/institution/Faculty
%20of%20Health%20Sciences/MB%20ChB%20Medicine/
Year%203%20Medicine%20and%20Surgery%20-
%20Hippocrates/ENT%20-%20ENT%20examination/index.
html

Eye examination:
https://www.youtube.com/watch?v=YqL6lMGE5os

Resuscitation Council (UK) (2021). Available at https://www.
resus.org.uk/library/2021-resuscitation-guidelines/adult-
basic-life-support-guidelines

5 Examination of the cardiovascular system

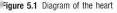

Figure 5.1 Diagram of the heart

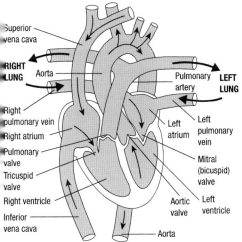

Superior vena cava

RIGHT LUNG

Aorta

Pulmonary artery

LEFT LUNG

Right pulmonary vein

Right atrium

Pulmonary valve

Tricuspid valve

Right ventricle

Inferior vena cava

Left atrium

Left pulmonary vein

Mitral (bicuspid) valve

Aortic valve

Left ventricle

Aorta

Source: Mary Miller, 2012, *Nursing & Health Survival Guide: Dental Nursing*, Pearson Education Limited; © Pearson Education Limited.

- The heart and circulatory system make up the cardiovascular system
- The heart works as a pump that pushes blood to the organs, tissues and cells of the body

DOI: 10.4324/9781003260325-6

- Blood delivers oxygen and nutrients to every cell and removes the carbon dioxide and waste products made by those cells
- Blood is carried from the heart to the rest of the body through a complex network of arteries, arterioles and capillaries
- Blood is returned to the heart through venules and veins
- An ABCDE assessment (Resuscitation Council (UK), 2021) may be needed before examination; the patient may be experiencing chest pain, so give analgesia at the earliest opportunity. It is important to rule out an emergency such as acute coronary syndrome
- Investigate the problem with a holistic health history; refer to Table 1.6
- Associated symptoms for exploration: breathlessness, chest pains, palpitations, syncope, nausea and/or vomiting, weakness or fatigue, leg pain or cramps, any swollen ankles, any weight gain/loss?
- Be aware of red flag markers: central crushing chest pain coming on at rest
- Look for environmental factors such as glyceryl trinitrate spray

■ EXAMINATION

General inspection

- General inspection of the hands: note clubbing, which may be indicative of cyanotic heart disease or subacute bacterial endocarditis (SBE)
- Note temperature – cold hands may indicate poor perfusion
- Look for Osler's nodes – red painful areas of infarction

- Look for splinter haemorrhages and nail bed infarcts seen in SBE
- Look for peripheral cyanosis; this may occur with or without central cyanosis and is more difficult to detect in dark skin
- Radial pulse: palpate the radial artery, feel both radial pulses for symmetry, assess rate, rhythm, regularity, character and volume. Use the tips of at least two or three fingers laid along the artery just above the wrist
- Blood pressure: measure on both arms. Consider checking blood pressure in lying and standing positions – a difference of 20 mmHg may indicate orthostatic hypotension
- *Note: A difference of 10–15 mmHg may indicate arterial compression or obstruction*
- Examine the face and upper body to note any breathlessness or use of accessory muscles

Examine the eyes

- Pale conjunctiva – SBE, anaemia, conjunctival pallor is a significant indication of anaemia regardless of skin colour
- Yellow deposits around eyes indicates xanthelasma – high cholesterol
- White rings around iris – corneal arcus, high cholesterol
- Icterus – jaundice

Examine the mouth

- Central cyanosis: a blue or grey discolouration of the facial skin and tongue and lips due to high levels of deoxygenated haemoglobin
- Lift tongue and inspect at base
- Look at palate – high arched palate in Marfan's syndrome

- Look at tongue – dehydration
- Inspect dentition

Examination of the jugular venous pulse (JVP)

There is no valve between the right heart and the large vessels supplying it, therefore the filling and contracting of the right atrium causes a pressure wave to travel back through the veins feeding it. This can be seen in the neck at the internal jugular vein.

- The patient should be in a supine position of 30–45°
- This is commonly used to assess the presence of right heart failure
- The vertical height of the internal jugular vein above the manubriosternal angle is measured – it starts between the two heads of the sternocleidomastoid and heads towards the angle of the jaw and the earlobe
- It should not be raised more than 3–4 cm

Figure 5.2 Measuring the height of the jugular venous pulse

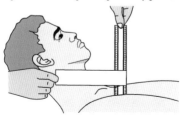

Note *If the JVP is not visible, press on the liver to raise*
the hepatojugular reflex; but be sure to release when
measuring the JVP.

Inspect the precordium

- Inspect the chest for scars and chest wall asymmetry

Palpation

- Palpate the apex beat – this is associated with the first
  heart sound and described as the point of maximal
  impulse. It lies at the fifth intercostal space in the
  midclavicular line. It may be seen normally in slim
  patients. In pathology, the apex deviates to the
  anterior axillary line and down in left ventricular
  hypertrophy
- Palpate for thrills (palpable murmur) and parasternal
  heave (right ventricular hypertrophy)

The areas for palpation are related to the anatomical
positions of the important cardiac structures in the chest:

- Aortic area – second intercostal space, right sternal
  border
- Pulmonary area – second intercostal space, left sternal
  border
- Tricuspid area – fourth intercostal space, left sternal
  border
- Apex/mitral area – fifth intercostal space, midclavicular
  line

Figure 5.3 Areas for palpation

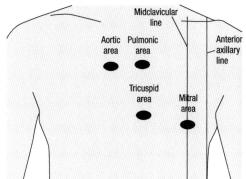

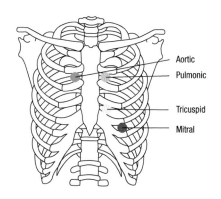

Auscultation

The diaphragm of the stethoscope is designed to pick up high-pitched sounds and the bell for low – remember di-high, bell-low! All areas of the heart need to be listened to with both the diaphragm and the bell.

Note *Ensure that you have familiarised yourself with the normal cardiac cycle of heart sounds.*

Figure 5.4 Atrioventricular and semilunar valves

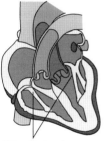

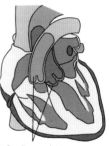

Atrioventricular valves

First heart sound, 'lub', occurs when atrioventricular valves close

Semilunar valves

Second heart sound, 'dup', occurs when semilunar valves close

Auscultate for heart sounds with the patient lying at an angle of 45°. The main areas to auscultate are:

- Aortic area
- Pulmonary area
- Tricuspid area
- Mitral area

Additional sounds:

- Third heart sound – rapid ventricular filling; can be normal under age of 30 or in pregnancy. Can be found in left ventricular fibrillation or fibrosed ventricle
- Fourth heart sound – always pathological; causes include left ventricular hypertrophy, hypertension and aortic stenosis

Auscultating for murmurs

Murmurs are when structural defects in the heart's chambers or valves cause turbulent blood flow. Detecting murmurs takes lots of practice:

- What does it sound like?
- Where is it loudest?
- To where does it radiate?
- Does the murmur occur in systole or diastole?

Types of murmur

- Systolic
- Diastolic
- Continuous

Position

Some murmurs are more easily heard when gravity aids the flow of blood on auscultation

Additional positioning of the patient for auscultation

- Place the patient in the left lateral position: listen to the tricuspid and mitral areas using the bell. This is the best position in which to detect mitral problems

- Ask the patient to sit forward and hold their breath: listen over the aortic and pulmonic valves and over the left sternal border using the diaphragm. This is a good position in which to detect aortic problems
- While the patient is in this position, listen to the lung bases to detect any crackles

Completing the cardiovascular examination

- Auscultate the aorta, renal and iliac arteries for bruits
- Use the bell and, when listening to the carotid, ask the patient to hold the breath
- Palpate all peripheral pulses
- Check for sacral and pedal oedema – right ventricular failure
- Check for skin arterial/venous insufficiency – hair loss, cyanosis, pallor, ulceration

Note A bruit is a whooshing sound caused by turbulent blood flow through a narrowed artery.

■ SUMMARY

A holistic history will guide the clinical examination and suggest a probable clinical diagnosis.

Always rule out life-threatening disease first. Exclude acute coronary syndrome with any chest pain.

Pain presentation may vary in women with nausea, lethargy and fatigue being significant symptoms. Knowledge of anatomy and physiology are key to understanding pathophysiology, for example, the apical impulse is non-palpable in approximately half of all adults.

■ **USEFUL RESOURCES**

Cardiovascular examination:

https://meded.ucsd.edu/clinicalmed/heart.htm; https://geekymedics.com/cardiovascular-examination-2/

Heart sounds:

https://www.easyauscultation.com/cases-Quiz?courseid=22

Measurement of the JVP:

https://www.youtube.com/watch?v=MZKSkVSbH8k

National Institute of Health and Clinical Excellence (2020). Acute Coronary Syndromes. Available at https://www.nice.org.uk/guidance/ng185

National Institute of Health and Care Excellence (2021) COVID-19 Rapid Guideline: Managing COVID-19. Available at https://www.nice.org.uk/guidance/ng191

Resuscitation Council (UK) (2021). Available at https://www.resus.org.uk/library/2021-resuscitation-guidelines/adult-basic-life-support-guidelines

6 Examination of the respiratory system

The respiratory system consists of nose, mouth, pharynx, larynx, trachea, bronchi, bronchioles and alveoli.

Figure 6.1 Respiratory system

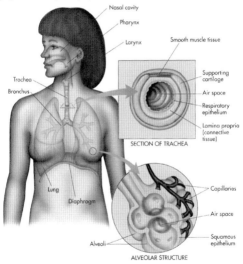

Nasal cavity

Pharynx

Larynx

Smooth muscle tissue

Trachea

Bronchus

Supporting cartilage

Air space

Respiratory epithelium

Lamina propria (connective tissue)

SECTION OF TRACHEA

Lung

Diaphragm

Capillaries

Air space

Alveoli

Squamous epithelium

ALVEOLAR STRUCTURE

Source: Mary Miller, 2012, *Nursing & Health Survival Guide: Dental Nursing*, Pearson Education Limited; © Pearson Education Limited.

DOI: 10.4324/9781003260325-7

These organs and tissues work together to ensure that oxygen is delivered to the bloodstream and carbon dioxide is removed. If you understand the basic structures of this system, it will help you to recognise any abnormalities.

Note *Extreme lung disease does not always produce clinical signs, e.g. silent chest in asthma.*

- An ABCDE assessment (Resuscitation Council (UK), 2021) may be needed before examination continues; the patient may be in acute respiratory distress
- Investigate the problem with a holistic health history (refer to Table 1.6)
- Associated symptoms to explore – breathlessness, wheeze, chest pain, ankle swelling, hoarseness, any weight changes, changes to sense of taste or smell, change in number of pillows used to sleep and cough. Is the cough productive? If so, colour and volume of sputum
- Be aware of red flag markers: haemoptysis, unintentional weight changes, night sweats, past history of cancers and nocturnal breathing difficulties disturbing sleep
- Look for environmental factors such as sputum and inhalers

■ EXAMINATION

General inspection

- General inspection of the hands – see Chapter 2 – note clubbing, peripheral cyanosis, splinter haemorrhages
- Test for capillary refill

- Note hand temperature: carbon dioxide retention or poor circulation
- Ask the patient to stretch their arms and hands in front of them for around 30 seconds to assess for fine tremor from overuse of bronchodilators or flapping tremor of CO_2 retention
- Take vital signs – temperature, pulse, respiration, blood pressure and oxygen saturation
- Examine the face and upper body to observe any breathlessness
- Observe pattern of respiration: pursed lips, breathlessness when talking, nasal flaring

Inspect the eyes

- Pale conjunctiva may indicate anaemia
- Suffusion may indicate CO_2 retention

Inspect the mouth

- Cyanosis – central, look under the tongue
- Dehydration from mouth breathing

Examine the lymph nodes

- Palpate the cervical, occipital, supraclavicular and axillae to detect any enlarged nodes – consider carcinoma of the bronchus

Examine the JVP (see Chapter 5)

- If raised, could indicate cor pulmonale or superior vena cava obstruction

Inspect the chest

Observe for:

- Scars or signs of surgery and symmetry of movement on respiration
- Chest shape and diameter – barrel chest from hyperinflation or pectus carinatum (pigeon chest) – sternum and costal cartilages are prominent and protrude from chest – consider rickets or asthma
- The rate, rhythm and depth of breathing – fast deep breaths consider anxiety – prolonged expiratory phase and pursed lipped breathing consider COPD
- Curvature of the spine – kyphosis or scoliosis

Figure 6.2 Curvature of the spine

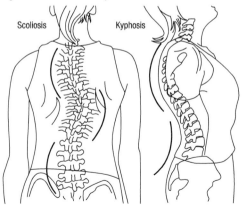

Palpation

- Palpate the trachea – feel the tracheal rings in the centre and a space on either side, if the trachea is not central, it may indicate a pneumothorax or tumour
- Locate and palpate the apex beat (see Chapter 5) – may be shifted to the left if the heart is enlarged, e.g. cor pulmonale
- Palpate the front and back of the chest wall for tenderness, crepitus, temperature, moisture, lumps and alignment, tenderness may be caused by trauma or pleurisy, pulled muscles or metastases
- Assess chest wall symmetry and expansion – place your hands symmetrically over each side of the lower chest with thumbs and fingers spread apart. Ask the patient to inspire deeply and watch the movement of your hands. It should be equal; if not, expansion may be decreased by consolidation, effusion, collapse or pneumothorax
- Palpate for tactile fremitus: this is a vibration felt on the surface of the chest as the patient speaks. Compare side to side at three or four levels. Place the ulnar edge of your palms on the chest and ask the patient to keep saying '99' loudly while you auscultate. Vibrations that are more intense on one side may indicate abnormalities such as consolidation

Percussion

- Percuss the chest to find the boundaries of the lungs and to find out whether they are filled with air, fluid or solid material

Figure 6.3 Assessing chest expansion and palpating for tactile fremitus

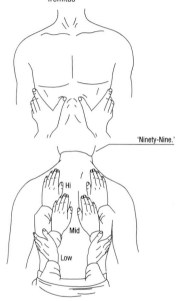

'Ninety-Nine.'

Hi

Mid

Low

Source: E. Diaz-Guzman, M.M. Budev, 2008, Accuracy of the physical examination in evaluating pleural effusion, *Cleveland Clinic Journal of Medicine*, 75: 297–303. Reprinted with permission; © Cleveland Clinic Foundation. All rights reserved.

- When percussing the back, ask the patient to cross their arms to move the scapula out of the way
- Percuss both sides of the chest and the top, middle and lower segments, begin at lung apices and continue in the intercostal spaces, make side-to-side comparisons
- You should hear normal resonant sounds: hyper-resonance indicates increased air, e.g. pneumothorax, emphysema. Dullness indicates decreased air, e.g. atelectasis, pneumonia. Flatness indicates highly consolidated areas, e.g. atelectasis, pleural effusion

Figure 6.4 Areas to auscultate and percuss the chest: posterior (a) and anterior (b) chest

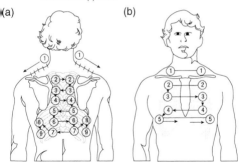

(a)   (b)

Auscultation

Before auscultation, review the anatomy of the lungs: the lower lobes occupy the bottom three-quarters of the posterior fields; the right middle lobe is heard in the right axilla, the lingula in the left axilla; the upper lobes are in the anterior chest and at the top one-quarter of the posterior fields.

Figure 6.5 Auscultation: LLL, left lower lobe; LUL, left upper lobe; RLL, right lower lobe; RML, right middle lobe; RUL, right upper lobe

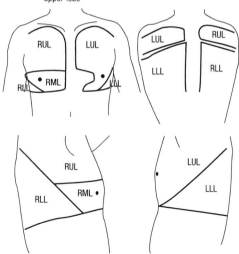

- As air moves through the bronchi, it creates sound waves that travel through the chest wall; these sounds alter over larger airways compared to smaller airways and also if they pass through fluid, mucus or narrowed airways
- You need to listen to top, middle, bottom and axilla on both sides for a full inspiration and expiration
- Ask the patient to breathe through their open mouth; make sure you are not listening over clothes. If a patient is excessively hairy, damp the hairs down

Note *When listening to the chest, you are ascertaining whether breath sounds are normal and whether there are any abnormal extra sounds.*

Normal breath sounds

- Bronchial – loud, high-pitched and discontinuous – heard only over upper trachea. If heard in other areas of the lung, consider consolidation
- Bronchovesicular – medium-pitched and continuous – heard near main bronchi
- Vesicular – soft and low-pitched (like wind through the trees) – heard in most of the lung fields

Abnormal breath sounds

- Crackles – intermittent non-musical crackling sounds that are caused by collapsed or fluid-filled alveoli popping open – can be coarse or fine
- Fine crackles – similar to the sound made by rubbing your hair through your fingers; occur in conditions such as pulmonary fibrosis, congestive cardiac failure and pneumonia

- Coarse crackles – like bubbling or gurgling as the air moves through secretions in the larger airways; consider COPD and pulmonary oedema
- Wheezes – continuous sounds, often high-pitched and heard first on expiration, caused by partially blocked airways. If the blockage becomes more severe, the wheeze may also be heard on inspiration. A wheeze may be found in asthma, bronchitis or obstruction from a tumour
- Stridor – a high-pitched crowing sound heard during inspiration that needs to be acted on immediately Causes include croup and obstruction by a foreign body
- Pleural friction rub – a low-pitched grating rubbing sound heard on inspiration and expiration caused by pleural inflammation, which sounds like 'crunching leaves', often accompanied by pain

Assess vocal fremitus

- Used to listen over an area where you suspect abnormal bronchial breathing to check for abnormal breath sounds. Ask the patient to repeat words as you listen with a stethoscope
- Bronchophony – ask the patient to say '99' repeatedly; if lung tissue is normal, sound is muffled; over consolidation sound unusually loud and clear

■ SUMMARY

Be systematic in your approach, inspect, palpate, percuss and auscultate. Maintain the patient's privacy and dignity, and ensure you clean your stethoscope. Remember to compare left to right and to examine the back and front of the chest to ensure that you have examined all of the lung fields. A good understanding of the underlying anatomy will help you to locate exactly where you locate any abnormal findings.

■ USEFUL RESOURCES

Lung sounds:
http://www.3m.com/healthcare/littmann/lung.html
https://geekymedics.com/jugular-venous-pressure-jvp/
Lung examination:
https://geekymedics.com/respiratory-examination-2/
https://meded.ucsd.edu/clinicalmed/lung.html
Resuscitation Council (UK) (2021). Available at https://www.resus.org.uk/library/2021-resuscitation-guidelines/adult-basic-life-support-guidelines

7 Examination of the abdominal system

The gastrointestinal system includes the mouth, pharynx, oesophagus, stomach, small intestine and large intestine. The accessory organs include the liver, pancreas, gallbladder, bile ducts and spleen.

Figure 7.1 Digestive system

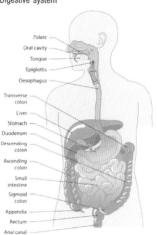

DOI: 10.4324/9781003260325-8

- An ABCDE assessment (Resuscitation Council (UK), 2021) may be needed before examination continues; the patient may be in acute abdominal pain so give analgesia at the earliest opportunity. It is important to rule out an emergency condition and assessment should focus on identifying patients with an acute abdomen that need urgent surgical referral and intervention, e.g. abdominal sepsis/peritonitis/intestinal obstruction and pancreatitis
- Be aware of verbal and non-verbal cues, e.g. grimacing and guarding
- Investigate the problem with a holistic health history; refer to Table 1.6
- Associated symptoms for exploration: pain, relationship to food, nausea and/or vomiting (describe vomit), change in bowel habit, urinary changes, dysphagia, weight loss or gain, any change in appetite, change in micturition, risk of pregnancy
- Be aware of red flag markers: change in bowel habit, blood in stools, urine or vomit, past history of cancer

■ EXAMINATION

Note *The abdomen is defined as the region lying between the thorax above (separated by the diaphragm) and the pelvic cavity below. The abdomen can be divided either into nine portions or simply four quadrants and three regions.*

General inspection

- General inspection of the hands: look at the nails for signs of leukonychia, which may indicate low albumin in

Figure 7.2 Parts of the abdomen

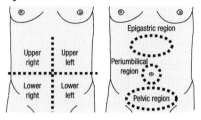

liver disease, koilonychia, which may indicate iron deficiency, clubbing, which may indicate inflammatory bowel disease, cirrhosis and coeliac disease in the abdominal system Look for peripheral cyanosis; this may occur with or without central cyanosis and is more difficult to detect in dark skin

- Note the palms – palmar erythema, a blotchy redness of the palms, may indicate chronic liver disease in the abdomen
- Examination for liver flap – this is similar to the flapping tremor of carbon dioxide retention (see Chapter 6). It is characteristic of encephalopathy if present

Inspect the eyes

- Sclera – note signs of jaundice and xanthelasma. Conjunctival pallor is a significant indication of anaemia regardless of skin colour

Inspect the mouth

- Note signs of angular stomatitis – a reddening of the corners of the mouth is a sign of vitamin B deficiency

- Dentition – signs of decay
- Inspect the tongue for thrush and glossitis
- Observe the breath: note hepatic foetor, a musty smell indicative of liver disease; alcohol; a sweet pear drop smell indicating ketosis

Palpate the supraclavicular nodes

- Observe for an enlarged isolated node on the left side (Virchow's node), which, if present, may indicate a gastric carcinoma

Examine the abdomen/chest wall

- Observe for spider naevi – telangiectatic capillary lesions with a central red area with capillaries spreading out from this. More than five may indicate liver disease
- Observe for gynaecomastia – excessive development of male mammary glands is often caused by liver disease

Examining the abdomen

- Before commencing, ask the patient if they would like to empty their bladder
- Ask the patient to report any pain and observe their face for non-verbal signs of pain
- Expose the patient from below the breast to the pubis
- If the patient can tolerate it, position supine with one pillow only, with their arms by their sides
- Auscultation is performed *before* percussion and palpation, as vigorously touching the abdomen may disturb the intestines, perhaps artificially altering their activity and thus bowel sounds

Inspection

Observe the abdomen for any scars.

Figure 7.3 Surgical incisions

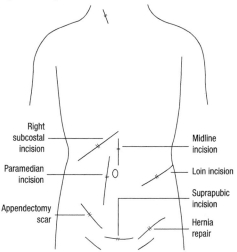

Right subcostal incision

Paramedian incision

Appendectomy scar

Midline incision

Loin incision

Suprapubic incision

Hernia repair

Ensure that you look both from the end of the bed and level with the patient's abdomen for distension – consider the 5 Fs:

- Fat
- Fluid

Faeces
- Foetus
- Flatus

Note *Always consider the possibility of pregnancy in women of childbearing age.*

- Observe for symmetry: any bulging may indicate a hernia
- Any obvious pulsations, which may indicate an aneurysm
- Any stomas
- Any bruising (ecchymosis) around the umbilicus – Cullen's sign
- Any bruising (ecchymosis) on the flanks, Grey Turner's sign, may indicate bleeding or pancreatitis

Note *Ecchymosis in dark skin may present as a purple or dark brown discolouration. Due to the increased melanin pigmentation, it might be difficult to see immediate bruising (which often appears red in light skin).*

Auscultation

- The bowel sounds can be assessed by lightly pressing the diaphragm of the stethoscope in the right lower quadrant

Note *As the bowel sounds are transmitted across the quadrants of the abdomen, you only need to listen in one quadrant unless the bowel sounds are absent. In this case, listening to each quadrant in turn is indicated.*

Classification of bowel sounds

- Normal bowel sounds – low-pitched, gurgling and intermittent
- High-pitched sounds – tinkling, indicative of subacute obstruction
- Borborygmus – very loud gurgling that can be heard without a stethoscope, indicative of diarrhoea or increased peristalsis
- Absent sounds – indicative of peritonitis or an ileus. You may need to listen for up to 5 minutes
- Listen for bruits with the bell of the stethoscope (see Chapter 5): just above the umbilicus slightly left of the midline for the aorta to detect aneurysm; either side of the midline just above the umbilicus for the renal arteries and the femoral arteries

Percussion

Percussion of the abdomen is a useful tool for discovering rebound tenderness, determining the size of enlarged organs and masses and defining shifting dullness

- You normally hear two sounds in the abdomen – tympany and dullness
- Tympany may be heard over air-filled organs like bowel and stomach
- Solid organs or masses produce a dull sound on percussion

Examining for ascites

Percussion can be quite helpful in determining the cause of abdominal distension, particularly in distinguishing between fluid (aka ascites) and gas. Assessment of shifting dullness – this method depends on the fact that air-filled intestines will float on top of any fluid that is present.

- Start percussing centrally, then move down laterally until dullness is detected
- Keep your finger on this spot and ask the patient to roll onto the side opposite to where the dullness has been detected
- After around 30 seconds with the patient in this position, repeat the percussion
- If the dullness was caused by fluid it will have moved by gravity from the marked spot and the original dull area will now be resonant

Palpation

- Palpation of the abdomen includes both light and deep palpation
- Before you begin the examination, ask the patient if they have any pain and start away from the pain
- Ask the patient to alert you if you cause any pain and observe for non-verbal signs of pain

Light palpation

This helps to assess the musculature in the abdomen for any surface abnormalities and tenderness. Using one hand, press down around 1–2 cm and make gentle rotating movements, flexing at the metacarpophalangeal joints, keeping the hand flat. The abdomen should be soft and not tender. If the patient experiences pain, ascertain whether it is more painful when pressure is applied or removed – rebound tenderness. Observe for involuntary tension in the abdominal muscles (guarding).

Deep palpation

To perform deep palpation, place one hand over the other, particularly in obese patients, and press down 5–7.5 cm. Follow the same clockwise pattern, rotating through the quadrants as you did for light palpation. If you feel a mass, describe its location, size, shape and whether it is pulsatile.

Note *Structures that may be felt in a normal abdomen:*

- *Lower pole of right kidney*
- *Abdominal aorta*
- *Caecal squelch*
- *Descending and/or sigmoid colon*
- *Uterus*
- *Bladder*

Note *Signs of peritonitis – rebound tenderness, involuntary guarding, absent bowel sounds and extreme pain on light palpation.*

■ EXAMINATION OF ABDOMINAL ORGANS

Percussion of the liver

Percuss both the upper and lower borders to determine the span of the liver:

- To identify the upper border, start percussing on the right side in the midclavicular line in an area of resonance until the note changes to dullness
- This may be difficult in women with large breasts. You can start percussion under the breast tissue

- To identify the lower border, start percussion in the right midclavicular line below the umbilicus and percuss up, from tympani to dullness
- Measure the span in centimetres. In an adult, the liver span is normally 6–12 cm

Palpation of the liver

The liver is hidden under the ribs so is not generally easily palpated:

Figure 7.4 Palpation of the liver

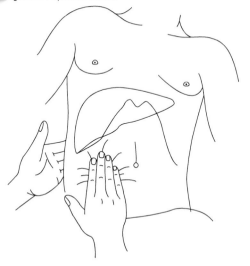

- Use the right hand positioned in the right iliac fossa with the fingers parallel to the costal margin
- Place your left hand underneath the patient's back approximately at the location of the liver
- Exert gentle pressure and ask the patient to take a deep breath. As the patient inhales, you may feel the liver slipping under the diaphragm
- Work upwards towards the ribs until the liver is palpated
- If you feel the liver edge it should be smooth; a cirrhotic liver may feel knobbly and tender
- The liver edge may be felt normally in slim patients and also in patients with a chest that is hyper-expanded, e.g. COPD

Note *Causes of an enlarged liver: alcohol, cancer, chronic liver disease and biliary obstruction.*

The spleen

The spleen is approximately the size of a clenched fist and is normally hidden underneath the left costal cartilages:

- If it is enlarged, this happens in a downward pattern extending towards the right iliac fossa and therefore it is necessary to start here to begin palpation
- In a technique similar to palpating the liver, the right hand is positioned in the right iliac fossa with the fingers pointing towards the left axilla
- The left hand reaches over to support the posterior lower rib cage. Ask the patient to breathe in and press inwards and upwards
- Work your way upwards with your right hand towards the left costal margin

igure 7.5 Palpation of the spleen

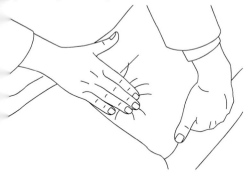

Note *Causes of a large spleen: portal hypertension secondary to cirrhosis, malaria, glandular fever and idiopathic thrombocytopenia.*

The kidneys

The kidneys are retroperitoneal, lying on either side of the vertebral column at the level of T12 and 13. The right kidney is displaced by the liver and lies a little lower than the left.

   You may be able to palpate the right kidney in a slim patient:

• Place the left hand underneath the patient in the right loin at the twelfth rib
• Place the right hand in the right upper quadrant above lateral and parallel to the rectus muscle

- Ask the patient to take a deep breath and, at the peak of inspiration, press your hands together in a duckbill fashion and try to capture the kidney between the two hands
- If the kidney is palpable, describe its size, shape and any tenderness

Figure 7.6 Palpation of the kidney

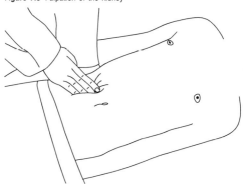

To palpate the left kidney, stand on the patient's left side and repeat the procedure with the left hand uppermost.

Note *Causes of a unilateral palpable kidney:*
hydronephrosis, acute pyelonephritis and carcinoma.
Causes of bilateral palpable kidneys: hydronephrosis,
polycystic disease and nephritic syndrome.

To complete the examination, a rectal examination and/or a vaginal examination may be indicated. If these are *not* performed, the fact must be documented.

SUMMARY

A holistic history will guide the clinical examination and suggest a probable clinical diagnosis therefore the importance of high-quality history and examination cannot be overestimated.

The severity of the abdominal pain does not always correspond with the severity of the condition.

Diagnosis is not delayed by the administration of analgesia, which is essential for patient comfort. If a patient is in extreme pain with a rigid abdomen, palpation may be unsafe and will not yield anything useful. In this case, direct referral to a senior team is the appropriate action.

■ USEFUL RESOURCES

Abdominal assessment:
https://www.youtube.com/watch?v=ufWO3pXygp4
https://geekymedics.com/abdominal-examination/
Association of Surgeons of Great Britain and Ireland (2014)
   Commissioning Guide: Emergency general surgery (acute abdominal pain). Available at https://www.rcseng.ac.uk/library-and-publications/rcs-publications/docs/emergency-general-guide/

National Institute of Health and Clinical Excellence (2020) Abdominal Aortic Aneurysm: Diagnosis and management. Available at https://www.nice.org.uk/guidance/ng156

Resuscitation Council (UK) (2021). Available at https://www.resus.org.uk/library/2021-resuscitation-guidelines/adult-basic-life-support-guidelines

8 Examination of the musculoskeletal system

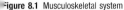

Figure 8.1 Musculoskeletal system

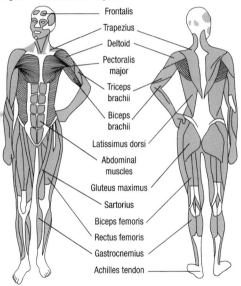

Frontalis
Trapezius
Deltoid
Pectoralis major
Triceps brachii
Biceps brachii
Latissimus dorsi
Abdominal muscles
Gluteus maximus
Sartorius
Biceps femoris
Rectus femoris
Gastrocnemius
Achilles tendon

The musculoskeletal system is made up of bones, muscles, joints, ligaments and tendons, and together they give the body its shape and structure. This system protects the

DOI: 10.4324/9781003260325-9

internal organs and provides the storage sites for minerals, and the bone marrow produces blood cells.

> *Note* *The principles of musculoskeletal examination are: LOOK, FEEL and MOVE, but some key points need to be addressed before completing a clinical examination.*

- You may need to complete an ABCDE assessment (Resuscitation Council (UK), 2021) and give analgesia before you can proceed with the examination
- Be safe – if the history or inspection indicates that further examination may be unsafe, stop and immobilise the affected area and seek expert help immediately
- All examinations stop at the point where there is gross deformity, loss of sensation or pain, and this should be documented
- Start the examination as soon as you see the patient – note gait, weight-bearing ability and how the patient is using the limbs as they approach you
- Be aware of verbal and non-verbal cues
- Investigate the problem with a holistic history; refer to Table 1.6
- Beware of distracting injuries; explore associated symptoms – unintentional weight loss, indirect trauma, nutritional status, victim of domestic or child abuse, systemic illness, change in bowel habit
- Remember that presenting with a musculoskeletal problem may be a manifestation of other systemic diseases

- Look for red flag markers: significant change from normal, loss of sensation and/or function, previous history of malignancy

◼ EXAMINATION

When examining the patient, compare left to right, and ensure that your examination does not add to the existing problem. Do not move to the next section of the examination if it endangers the health of the limb. The method used is 'look, feel and then move'.

Look/inspection

Look at all aspects of the area and note any of the following:

- Deformity – may indicate fracture or dislocation, congenital deformity, previous trauma, rheumatoid arthritis
- Swelling – may indicate trauma, infection
- Redness – may indicate infection
- Position – in relation to body, may indicate congenital deformity
- Wounds – old or new, signs of surgery
- Size of joint – in relation to normal, may indicate arthritis

Feel/palpation

Palpate all the muscles, bones, bony prominences and joints from the joint above to the joint below the affected area. Note any of the following:

- Areas of tenderness or crepitus – this may indicate fractures or tendon/ligament problems

- Establish the neurovascular status – check pulses, venous return and sensation distal to the problem area

Move

Compare left to right the full range of:

- Active movements – those that the patient can do themselves, which may be limited by pain
- Passive movements – those that you can take the limb through; this range will be greater than active movement and will assess the integrity of the tendons and ligaments
- Resisted movements – movements made against an opposing force to check equality of strength. Inequality may indicate a neurological problem

Description of range of movements

Table 8.1 Description of range of movements

ACTION	MOVEMENT	EXAMPLE
Flexion	Decreasing the joint angle, bending	Elbow, knee
Extension	Increasing the joint angle, straightening	Elbow, knee
Abduction	Movement away from the midline	Shoulder, hip
Adduction	Movement towards the midline	Shoulder, hip
Circumduction	Involves all elements allowing a circular motion	Shoulder, thumb

Table 8.1 (*Continued*)

ACTION	MOVEMENT	EXAMPLE
Retraction	Moving backward	Jaw
Protraction	Moving forward	Jaw
Pronation	Turning downward	Forearm
Supination	Turning upward	Forearm
Internal rotation	Rotating toward the midline	Shoulder, hip
External rotation	Rotating away from the midline	Shoulder, hip
Inversion	Turning inward	Ankle
Eversion	Turning outward	Ankle

Normal range of joint movements

Table 8.2 Normal range of joint movements

JOINT	MOVEMENT
Temporomandibular	Retraction, protraction, open and close mouth
Cervical spine	Flexion, extension, lateral movements, rotation
Thoracic spine	Flexion, extension, lateral movements, rotation
Lumbar spine	Flexion, extension, lateral movements, rotation

(*Continued*)

Table 8.2 (*Continued*)

JOINT	MOVEMENT
Shoulder	Flexion, extension, abduction, adduction, internal and external rotation
Elbow	Flexion, extension, pronation, supination
Wrist	Flexion, extension, radial and ulnar deviation
Fingers	Flexion, extension, abduction, adduction
Thumb	Flexion, extension, abduction, adduction, opposition
Hip	Flexion, extension, abduction, adduction, internal and external rotation
Knee	Flexion, extension
Ankle	Flexion, extension, inversion, eversion
Toes	Flexion, extension, abduction, adduction

■ SUMMARY

A holistic history will be the key to diagnosis. Listen carefully to the exact mechanism of injury and development of pain and symptoms, as these should guide your examination. Remember that not all presenting cases have

rauma-related issues and their condition may be an
ndicator of systemic disease. In assessing the severity of
he problem pain scoring is useful, but also explore how the
condition is affecting the patient's activities of daily living.

Always compare both sides, examine the less painful
side first as this gives a start point. Use the 'look, feel,
move' method and do not to proceed with the examination
f there is the potential of causing a worsening of the
condition.

■ USEFUL RESOURCES

Clinical examination:
https://geekymedics.com/category/osce/clinical-
    examination/msk/
Musculoskeletal health:
https://www.gov.uk/government/publications/
    musculoskeletal-health-applying-all-our-health/
    musculoskeletal-health-applying-all-our-health
Purcell, D. (2016) *Minor Injuries: A clinical guide*, 3rd edn.,
    Edinburgh, Elsevier.
Resuscitation Council (UK) (2021). Available at https://www.
    resus.org.uk/library/2021-resuscitation-guidelines/adult-
    basic-life-support-guidelines

9 Examination of the nervous system

The nervous system is divided into parts: the central nervous system (CNS), which includes the brain and the spinal cord, and the peripheral nervous system (PNS), which includes the cranial nerves and the peripheral nerves. This system can be difficult to assess as the presenting symptoms may be organic or psychological in origin, which may be problematic to differentiate. The examiner must consider the three Ds: dementia, delirium or depression as causes for symptoms. This section does not cover a mental state examination but, rather, focuses on the physical examination skills. For a comprehensive examination, a clear holistic history is vital, and it may be necessary to complete a mental state examination in conjunction with a physical examination. A cranial nerve examination may be needed, but this is beyond the scope of this book and, if needed, referral to a specialist would be recommended.

- An ABCDE assessment (Resuscitation Council (UK), 2021) may be needed before examination continues
- Neurological presentations may be an indicator of underlying systemic disease
- Be aware of verbal and non-verbal cues
- Investigate the problem with a holistic health history; refer to Table 1.6
- Explore any associated symptoms: unintentional weight changes, vomiting, nausea, changes from normal
- Be aware of red flag markers: sudden-onset headache, change in vision, hearing, taste, fits, character/mood changes
- History may need corroboration with other people

DOI: 10.4324/9781003260325-10

◀ ABBREVIATED NEUROLOGICAL EXAMINATION

Table 9.1 Abbreviated neurological examination

ACTION	RATIONALE
General assessment	
Introduce yourself, ask the name and age of the patient, explain the procedure and request consent. Throughout, observe: general condition, weight loss, cyanosis, pallor, standard of self-care, orientation, confusion, memory loss, speech, facial expression and symmetry, ability to move face and limbs, abnormal movements, gait (in clinical situation, observe as patient walks in)	Assess general health: inaccurate data, slow or inappropriate answers, and being unkempt may indicate mental illness or dementia. Difficulty in articulating words (dysarthria) may indicate stroke, motor neurone disease, multiple sclerosis or cerebellar disease. Difficulty in understanding speech or using incorrect words (receptive or expressive dysphasia) may indicate stroke Lack of expression may indicate Parkinson's disease Loss of symmetry of the face at rest or on movement, is lower motor neuron weakness of the facial nerve (Bell's palsy – all of one side

(Continued)

Table 9.1 (*Continued*)

ACTION	RATIONALE
	of face) or upper motor neuron weakness (stroke – lower part of one half of the face)
	Lack of movement of one arm and/or leg may be due to stroke (upper motor neuron) or peripheral nerve lesion (lower motor neuron)
	Tremor may be due to Parkinson's disease, benign essential tremor, alcohol, drugs, etc.
	Dystonic movements may be drug-induced (metoclopramide, psychotropics)
Wash hands	To maintain infection control
With the patient sitting	
Check size, shape and symmetry of pupils and their direct and consensual reactions to light	Eye disease affects the size and shape of the pupil (e.g. iritis, glaucoma)
	Abnormal size of pupils may be due to drugs or damage to the optic cranial

ble 9.1 (*Continued*)

ACTION	RATIONALE
	nerve (II), the oculomotor cranial nerve (III) or the brain (especially trauma), rarely congenital Reduced or slow response to light may be congenital or caused by retinal, optic nerve or brain disease
Check eye movements with the head held still, asking patient to report any double vision	Squint, damage to cranial nerves III, IV or VI Nystagmus may be due to disease of the inner ear, cerebellum or pathways in the lower part of the brain
Shielding the opposite eye with a hand held along the nose and, after warning the patient, gently blow onto each eye, observing the blink response	This tests reflex pathway of sensation (upper division of trigeminal cranial nerve, V) and motor response (facial nerve, VII)
Ask patient to stand	Difficulty standing without pushing up with arms may indicate proximal muscle weakness (e.g. polymyalgia

(*Continued*)

Table 9.1 (*Continued*)

ACTION	RATIONALE
	rheumatica, steroids, alcohol)
With the patient standing	
While reassuring the patient that you will not let them fall and demonstrating this by the position of your arms just behind their shoulders, ask them to shut their eyes and stand still	Unsteadiness with eyes open indicates disease of the inner ear, cerebellum or pathways in the lower part of the brain. Unsteadiness only with eyes closed (positive Romberg's test) indicates difficulty with position sense (proprioception) which may result from severe B12 deficiency, syphilis and other disorders affecting the proprioception pathways in the posterior part of the spinal cord
With eyes still closed, ask the patient to hold out both hands with palms upwards	This is a very sensitive indicator of upper motor neuron weakness, usually due to stroke. The hand drifts so the palm turns inward and/or the hand drops

ble 9.1 (*Continued*)

CTION	RATIONALE
Vith eyes closed and rms still outstretched, ently touch one index nger and ask the patient to touch their nose with that finger. Repeat on the other side	This is a good screening test of sensation (e.g. peripheral neuropathy), motor function (e.g. stroke), position sense (especially diabetic peripheral neuropathy) and coordination (e.g. cerebellar or cerebellar pathway damage in multiple sclerosis)
Gait	
Ask the patient to walk: normally across the room to return on tiptoe to cross the room touching toe to heel in a straight line to return, walking on heels	Look for the shuffling, festinant gait of Parkinson's disease (running after one's centre of gravity) Walking, especially on toes or heels, tests leg power better than any bed-or chair-based-test Look for signs of upper motor neuron (spastic – increased tone) weakness due to stroke (weak stiff leg, difficulty supporting weight, especially on toe or

(*Continued*)

Table 9.1 (*Continued*)

ACTION	RATIONALE
	heel) or other diseases (motor neurone disease, multiple sclerosis). Also look for flaccid lower motor neuron weakness, e.g. foot drop owing to sciatic nerve root lesion (prolapsed disc), or peripheral nerve damage (peroneal nerve) Coordination (cerebellum and its pathways) and balance (inner ear and pathways) are stressed by heel–toe walking and by walking on toes and heels. Lesions in these areas are most likely due to demyelination (multiple sclerosis)
With the patient sitting again	
Ask the patient to hold out hands, dorsiflexed at wrist, 'stopping traffic', and ask them to resist your pressure to push	A sensitive indicator of upper motor neuron damage due to stroke Another sensitive indicator

ble 9.1 *(Continued)*

CTION	RATIONALE
ne fingers down flat est power of lorsiflexion and eversion f feet: 'stop me pushing your feet down' 'push my hands apart'	of upper motor neuron damage due to stroke
Compare tendon reflexes side to side: biceps triceps patellar ankle	Reflexes are exaggerated on the side affected by stroke or other upper motor neuron lesions They may be reduced with lower motor neuron pathology. This rarely affects arm reflexes but commonly occurs with disc lesions, affecting L5–S1 (ankle reflex reduced) and, less often, L3–4 or L4–5 (knee reflex reduced)
Wash hands	To maintain infection control
Testing sensation	
This is only necessary in comprehensive formal nervous system examinations and in the	To assess degree of diabetic peripheral neuropathy

(Continued)

Table 9.1 (*Continued*)

ACTION	RATIONALE
routine examination of patients with diabetes. Use monofilament for light touch and a tuning fork for vibration sense	

■ SUMMARY

Neurological presentations are notoriously difficult to assess as the symptoms may have an organic and/or psychological origin. A clear and comprehensive history is vital in assessing these clients and the practitioner should be holistic in their approach. Identifying red flag markers and any changes from the patient's normal health and cognitive status should prompt the practitioner to explore in greater depth. An abbreviated neurological clinical examination may be a good starting point and any anomalies discovered will support a referral to a specialist.

■ USEFUL RESOURCES

Clinical examination:
https://geekymedics.com/category/osce/clinical-examination/
    neuroosce/
https://geekymedics.com/cranial-nerve-exam/
Cognitive assessment tools:
https://www.alz.org/professionals/health-systems-clinicians/
    clinical-resources/cognitive-assessment-tools

ller, G. (2019) *Neurological Examination Made Easy*, 6th edn., Edinburgh, Elsevier.

suscitation Council (UK) (2021). Available at https://www.resus.org.uk/library/2021-resuscitation-guidelines/adult-basic-life-support-guidelines

10 Documentation of findings

- The notes that are made to document the findings are a record of the patient assessment, illness and treatment and are the only record of your actions
- Everything that is done should be recorded, including any discussions around findings or treatment with relatives or the patient
- Many areas have proformas for health assessment; if this is not the case, there are no specific rules about how assessments are documented. Generally, however, write up the assessment in the order in which the history and examination was conducted
- Diagrams may be useful when describing examination findings, e.g. drawing lungs to indicate areas dull to percussion
- Be cautious regarding the use of abbreviations and refer to policy in the area in which you are practising, in addition to your regulatory body's guidelines on documentation
- Ensure patient confidentiality is maintained and that local or national guidance is followed especially in relation to electronically held records

Note Some common abbreviations are used in this chapter but, when in doubt – write it out!

■ KEY POINTS

- Always record your name, signature and date, findings and management plan on every entry to the case notes

DOI: 10.4324/9781003260325-11

Record objective findings, abnormal findings and pertinent negatives
Notes need to be timely and legible

Note Patient notes are confidential; details should only be shared with professionals directly involved in the patient's care. Patients have a right to see their notes if they wish.

DEMOGRAPHIC DETAILS

Record

The patient's name, preferred form of address, date of birth, gender at birth
National Health ID number
Source of referral
GP details
Source of history, e.g. patient or carer
Date and time of examination

Presenting complaint (PC)

Document the major problem in one or two of the patient's own words, followed by duration, e.g. 'Feels like an elephant sat on my chest for the last hour'
- Do not use medical terminology
- Document any chronological symptoms, e.g. chest pain 2 hours, breathlessness 1 hour, dizziness 30 min

History of presenting complaint (HPC)

- Document onset, nature and course of each symptom
- Omit irrelevant details

- Put important patient comments in inverted commas
- Include other parts of history if relevant, e.g. smoking or family illness

Past history (PH)

- Document in chronological order
- Include important negatives, e.g. in patient with chest pain ask re previous MI, angina, hypertension, diabetes
- Document whether the patient has had any surgery or mental illness and exclude the common medical conditions (see Table 1.4)

Drug history (DH)

- Document the patient's medication, including prescribed, over-the-counter (OTC), recreational, homeopathic or herbal, borrowed, from other sources such as the Internet
- Record any adverse drug reactions prominently
- Record any compliance/concordance issues

Allergies

- Record any allergies to drugs, environment and food, their severity and any treatment needed

Family history (FH)

- Record age and current health or causes of death, and their ages of parents, siblings and children
- Record any evidence of common familial diseases, e.g. diabetes, stroke, hypertension, epilepsy

cial history (SH)

cord your findings from the history in these areas:

Occupation – past and current

Marital status

Living circumstances – accommodation

Social support

Financial situation

Hobbies

Belief system

Alcohol usage – past and present

Smoking habits – past and present

Recreational drug use – past and present

Sexual health history

ctivities of daily living (ADLs)

ecord your findings and document any change in:

Appetite and diet

Weight

Elimination

Mood

Exercise and sleep

Systematic enquiry (SE) or review of systems (ROS)

Document positive responses that are not explored in he HPC:

- HEENT – head, eyes, ears, nose, throat
- CVS – cardiovascular system
- RS – respiratory system
- GI – gastrointestinal

- GU – genitourinary (reproductive)
- PVS – peripheral vascular system
- ES – endocrine system
- MSS – musculoskeletal system
- CNS – central nervous system
- PSY – psychiatric

■ PROVISIONAL DIAGNOSIS (DDx)

Document

- Diagnoses that are supported by the history
- List in the order of probability

■ PLAN OF CARE OR TREATMENT PLAN (Rx)

Document

- Any immediate treatment
- Clinical examinations that need to be undertaken
- Information that has been discussed with the patient
- Any information that needs to be clarified or confirmed
- Any investigations needed to support or refute DDx
- Any results of investigations already known

■ DOCUMENTATION OF PHYSICAL EXAMINATION

General/ (on examination)

- Document a statement to describe the physical appearance, e.g. frail, drowsy, breathless, mental state, nutritional status

Record the findings of your general assessment: hands, mouth and eyes, presence of lymph nodes

DOCUMENT THE VITAL SIGNS

Record baseline vital signs: temperature (T), pulse (P) – nature and regularity, blood pressure (BP), capillary refill time (Cap refill), oxygen saturation (O_2 sats), height (HT), weight (WT)

CARDIOVASCULAR SYSTEM

Document findings of:

Jugular venous pressure (JVP) – height and character
Presence or absence of ankle oedema
Apex beat (AB) position, character, any thrills
Character and location of any cardiac thrills
Heart sounds (HS) – any added sounds or murmurs and grade
Peripheral pulses (PPs) – presence and strength
Presence of any bruits

RESPIRATORY SYSTEM

Document findings of:

- Presence of any chest wall deformity
  Jugular venous pressure (JVP) – height and character
- Trachea position – central or deviated
- Expansion and symmetry of respiration
- Percussion (PN) – any abnormality
- Breath sounds (BS) – added sounds and site
- Vocal resonance (VR) – site of abnormality

■ GASTROINTESTINAL SYSTEM

Document findings of:

- Mouth – own teeth, any abnormality with tongue or mucous membranes
- Abdomen – describe or draw scars, shape, hernias, tenderness and guarding, masses
- Enlargement of liver, kidneys or spleen (LKKS)
- Presence and extent of any ascites
- Bowel sounds (BS) – presence and nature
- Rectal examination (PR) done or not – findings
- Vaginal examination (VE) done or not – findings
- Men: external genitalia

■ MUSCULOSKELETAL SYSTEM

Document findings of:

- Gait and weight bearing
- Muscle or soft tissue changes
- Location of any swelling, colour, heat and tenderness, crepitus
- Deformities in joints
- Range of movements

■ CENTRAL NERVOUS SYSTEM

Document findings of:

- Results of any cognitive test
- Conscious level – AVPU or GCS
- Speech pattern – any abnormalities
- Cranial nerve examination if undertaken, including fundoscopy

Pupil – size and reaction to light (pupils equal and reacting to light, accommodating, PEARLA)

Motor, cerebellar, sensory reflexes: upper limb (UL), lower limb (LL), knee (K), biceps (B), triceps (T), supinator (S), plantar (PL), no abnormality detected (NAD)

DIFFERENTIAL DIAGNOSIS (Dx) and plan of care (Rx)

Record your conclusions and the most likely diagnoses in order of probability

If multiple pathology exists, make a problem list with key issues first

List investigations required

If a result is available, record it; if advice is needed, document this

Record any immediate management or treatment instigated

Document information given to the patient and family member

Document any diagnosis not discussed

Document the patient's concerns or fears

PROGRESS NOTES

- Date and sign all entries
- Record any unexpected change in the patient's condition

SUMMARY

Clear, concise and timely documentation of your consultation allows others in the multidisciplinary team to know what has happened to the patient. Pertinent negatives are as important as findings and means that the patient may not have to repeat the same information to several different health professionals. These notes may be called on at any time to examine the care received by the patient, consider what information you would need to continue the care for a patient; this is what should be in a set of case notes.

■ USEFUL RESOURCES

https://www.bfwh.nhs.uk/onehr/wp-content/uploads/2019/
11/5-Generic-Clinical-Record-Keeping-Standards-and-
Good-Practice-Handout.pdf

https://www.hcpc-uk.org/standards/meeting-our-standards/
record-keeping/

https://www.medicalprotection.org/uk/articles/an-mps-
essential-guide-to-medical-records